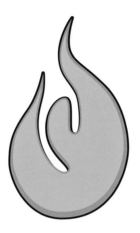

Speaking the Language of Miracles®

Learn how your words are the most powerful language you have.

Learn how this principle applies in every aspect of your life.

DEANNA SCOTT

Testimonials

" There are books that come along every now and then, which give you a jolt! Well, I've found it and I want everyone I know to have a copy of Speaking the Language of Miracles. This is more than a book, it is a lifestyle that can change a generation. I encourage you to read it, teach it, share it, and most importantly live it and watch what happens. You will discover that the rest of your life will be the best of your life. "
Simon T. Bailey
Author of Shift Your Brilliance: Harness the Power of You

"In life, all of us will experience challenges, circumstances and situations that will seem insurmountable. In her book, Deanna Scott provides hope, inspiration and practical ways we can experience victory over our adversity. "
Dermot Buffini
CEO of Buffini & Company

"*Speaking the language of Miracles* is a game changer. In business, our new approach is: everything is just a situation. Whether out of distress or an opportunity. We're moving forward towards the positive outcome in an instant. "
J. Lennox Scott
Chairman and CEO of John L. Scott Real Estate

"Read this book. What a wake up call! It helped me see through all my 'situations', in business and in life. I learned to recognize a lack of perspective and clarity. What an awesome and powerful guide you have in your hands. *Speaking the Language of Miracles* taught me to live in the now... Now! "
Ben Medina
Creative Director of Good Kingdom Group

"I absolutely loved reading this book. It's ability to cause you to reflect on your life and allow you to be inspired by your own future is truly amazing. I found myself in deep gratitude about every area of my life, knowing that I can turn it into whatever I choose to be. It's always the greatest gift to reflect from a place of empowerment, and you totally allow your reader to do that."

Ashley Norris
Yoga and Spiritual Lifestyle Instructor

" This book is invaluable for all aspects of your life. It is a working template for being in the now and utilizing the ancient wisdom of the vibratory force of our words to create our world. Read this book and ignite the divine spark with you and watch the magic happen in your life and the ones you love."

Brad Norris
Owner of Malibu Health Club & Spiritual Healer

" To say I love this book is an understatement! *Speaking The Language of Miracles* is truly a gift. This book is captivating, riveting and I truly could not put it down. I immediately bought it for family and friends, facing major health and life challenges. With 3o years of experience in organizational development, and the study of managerial excellence, and as a former director of training for two of Washington State's largest agencies, I have spent thousands of hours training and consulting with groups & individuals to empower them towards excellence. The key has always been to: affirm the desired end result. As it says in the book "whatever you think; you create." This book answered that need beautifully. Enjoy your read... It may change your life!"

Gail D. Swanson
Former Director of Training
Washington State Employment Security Department
Washington State Department of Social and Health Services

Table of Contents

Your Gifts Are Inside of You

I am here to show you how your language is one of the most powerful gifts that you have in this universe. This approach to wellness is best summarized in one powerful statement:

REMEMBER: THE ILLNESS IS NOT WHO YOU ARE.

If you are a parent whose child is fighting for his or her life, you are no longer alone. Deanna's amazing book has been put in your path just when you need it the most.

An old proverb says, "To know the road ahead, ask those coming back."

Deanna has been to the brink with her son - they have come back to help other parents and their children."

Editor - Ben Medina

TWENTY PERCENT (20%) OF THE NET PROCEEDS FROM BOOK SALES GOES DIRECTLY TO SUPPORT CHILDREN'S HOSPITALS.

speakingthelanguageofmiracles.com

LEARN HOW YOU CAN APPLY SPEAKING THE LANGUAGE OF MIRACLES IN EVERYTHING YOU DO.

- To Walk in the Positive Outcome you need to remember one thing:

THE SITUATION IS NOT WHO YOU ARE.[R]

- Learn how powerful your language is and what you are telling yourself.

- Learn how to be successful in business using the the Language of Miracles in the corporate world.

- Learn how to instill the Language of Miracles into our kids for the future.

- Learn how to make the right choices.

- Learn how to walk in the outcome.

- Learn how to NOT walk in the situation.

- When you use Language of Miracles, every day, you walk in the intent of the outcome you want to achieve.

- What's inside of you is much greater than the situation.

- Learn to walk in your God-given gifts.

CHAPTER

01

Health

YOUR LIFE CAN CHANGE IN AN INSTANT

YOUR
LIFE...

...Can change in an instant.

The story I wish to share is about my son, Brandon. Through his experience, Language of Miracles was born. Creating an intense path of revelation and reflection, offering the ability to access the incredible power we all have with our own language to better our lives.

WE can be the enduring change for our own miracles.

THIS IS BRANDON'S WALK

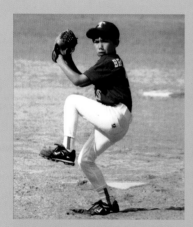

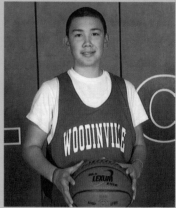

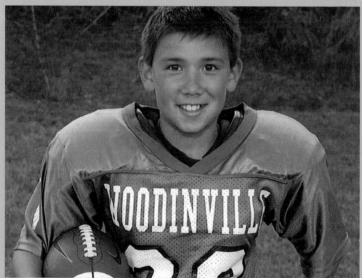

Brandon's Story
When he was ten years old...

On Mother's Day, May 10th, 2005, my family and I celebrated my son, Brandon's baseball tournament by playing a round of golf together. The following morning, Brandon was not feeling well and rather than go to school, I followed an inner impulse to take him to the doctor. It was uncharacteristic for me to take him to the doctor because I typically observe my kid's cold or flu symptoms over a course of a couple of days before visiting a doctor's office. Keep in mind, Brandon was always the healthiest member of our family and rarely ever came down sick. He was known as an outstanding athlete, who excelled at baseball, football and basketball.

The doctor thought Brandon had a common cold, but because recently, he had seen several cases of mononucleosis, he took the precaution of performing a blood test. Without that blood test my son would not be here today.

Two hours following the doctor visit, I received a call from the doctor telling me to rush Brandon to Seattle Children's Hospital based on the results showing an extremely low white blood cell count. Seattle Children's Hospital performed an emergency blood transfusion upon his arrival. The doctor told me Brandon was in a rare situation, and was diagnosed with an acute form of leukemia. The doctor shared he would not be leaving the hospital any time soon.

Brandon's first question was, "Mom, does this mean I'm going to die?" I told him, "the illness is not who you are."

And that is how our journey began.

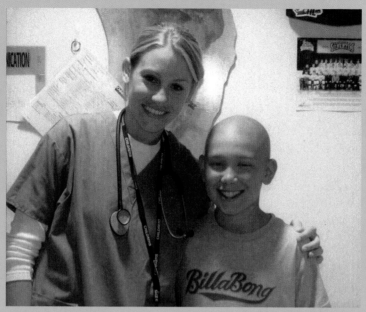

Brandon's nurse, Stacy

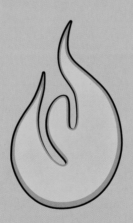

REMEMBER: THE ILLNESS IS NOT WHO I AM®

Brandon's Miracles

OUR MIRACLES WERE IN OUR LANGUAGE, WHAT WE SAID, WE CREATED. BRANDON'S MIRACLES WERE IN HIS LANGUAGE. WHAT HE SAID, HE CREATED.

For eight months, we witnessed miracles daily. The first miracle was when the doctor asked to do a blood test on Brandon, even though the doctor suspected a common cold. Without that blood test my son would not have been alive the next day.

The next miracle was when we got the blood test back in two hours. The doctor said it wouldn't be back for two or three days. After leaving the doctor's office, I asked Brandon if he wanted to go with me to take care of his sister's horse. His sister's horse was stabled in a rural area where there was never any cell service.

The next miracle — the phone rang and Brandon replied "that's weird, you never get cell service here." When I picked up the phone the doctor, in a panic, said: "Deanna it's an emergency, get Brandon to Seattle Children's hospital immediately, they are waiting for your arrival."

Right then I hung up the phone to call my husband, but there was no cell service.

Just to let you know how serious Brandon's illness was, the nurses were required to draw his blood to monitor his blood cells every hour on the hour for eight months. Brandon was throwing up blood every day, sometimes buckets of blood. I forgot how many blood transfusions that he had! His fevers of 106 degrees would sometimes last for three days. Brandon's temperature would not go down until he declared out loud "my temperature is 98.6," and visualized his temperature going down, and then it would. We would pray, but it would not change until he spoke faith upon himself.

When his temperature climbed to 106, he was taken to the intensive care unit.

The doctors shared how they were going to do a tracheotomy so he could breathe better. Right then I asked Brandon to focus on his temperature going down and that's when we saw it lowering.

They did not do the tracheotomy. Another miracle. What he said, he created. We witnessed so much power in his word. Every single day was a fight for his life. However, we never walked in the illness. Every day we reminded Brandon of who he was and spoke of his future, never speaking of his illness.

REMEMBER:
THE ILLNESS IS NOT WHO I AM®

Every Day that Brandon was Alive was a Miracle

Brandon's doctor told us that because of the type of Leukemia that Brandon had, he was going to need a bone marrow transplant. No one in the family was a match for Brandon. They put Brandon under anesthesia and went into his bone marrow to see what type he would need. Right before he went under he wrote out on paper: "I have healthy blood cells throughout my body and I am a healthy child of God" — over and over again on three pages. When the doctors came back to us, they shared that they had never seen this before with this type of Leukemia, that it was a miracle: "We are happy to share that your son does not need a bone marrow transplant. He has a higher chance of living." Tears of joy came running down our faces, thanking God.

When Brandon was able to write, he would write out his affirmations. That way we were walking in the intent of his affirmation that day, and we consistently witnessed miracles. This is in your language — whatever you say you create. So, make it positive. All we did was let Brandon shine. By not bringing up the illness, we spoke Faith upon him. When all of his friends and our family would come up to me and say: "Deanna, I don't know if I can go into Brandon's room and not cry," all I did was remind everyone: the illness is not my son, remember who Brandon was before the illness. Then everyone was walking in the outcome of Brandon leaving the hospital and not walking in the illness. They remembered Brandon as who he was before he got sick.

I AM WITH YOU

ALL
THE
WAY

Learning the Language of Miracles®

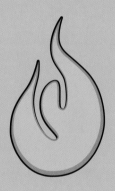

REMEMBER: THE ILLNESS IS NOT WHO I AM®

Wellness

I am here to share how your language is one of the most powerful gifts that you have in this universe. Do not let your words limit you. Whatever you say, you create, so make the distinctions between what you are saying and what you are telling yourself. Is it positive or negative?

Remember that the illness is not who you are and that you are the creator of your life. Create a life that you Love. Dream Big. Don't let setbacks hold you down. Continue to reinvent yourself. And remember: our best days are ahead of us.

If you have been told you have an illness, I hope this section of Wellness helps you. This was Brandon's walk and he proved to be a powerful being and a cancer survivor.

Parents

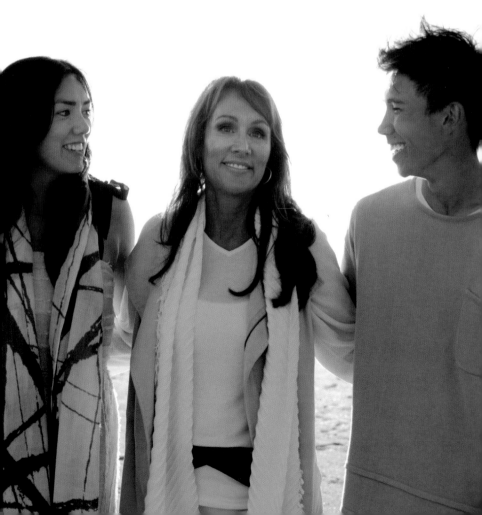

Parents can share this concept with their children by talking to them about having goals and dreams. By doing this, you can help your child reinvent himself/herself. Whenever bad situations occur, you can let your children know that it is just a situation and not who they are. You can teach them to walk in their own spirit and not get caught up in the situations they might find themselves in.

ACTIONS OF LOVE

Teach the Language of Miracles to family, friends, community members, hospital staff, and whoever your child sees.

1. Remind everyone that the illness is not your child, it's just the situation—it's not who they are

2. Walk in the positive outcome and remember who they were before they had the illness. Speak faith upon them

3. Your child is not the illness

4. Do not own the illness

5. And know... The Doctors are walking in solutions.

- [ ] VISUALIZE THE OUTCOME OF A HEALTHY CHILD

- [ ] ALWAYS FOCUS ON THE POSITIVE OUTCOME OF YOUR CHILD BEING HEALTHY, NOT THE ILLNESS

- [ ] IF YOU FOCUS ON THE ILLNESS, IT PERSISTS

- [ ] NEVER TELL YOUR CHILD HOW SICK THEY ARE, THE ILLNESS IS JUST A SITUATION

- [ ] INTERACT WITH YOUR CHILD IN THE SAME WAY YOU DID BEFORE HE/SHE GOT SICK

- [ ] EVEN IF YOUR SON/DAUGHTER HAS AN ILLNESS, DO NOT CHANGE THE WAY YOU PLAY AND TALK WITH HIM/HER

- [ ] REPLACE THE HOSPITAL ROOM ENVIRONMENT WITH YOUR HOME ENVIRONMENT

- [ ] BRANDON HAD PICTURES OF HIMSELF PLAYING FOOTBALL, BASEBALL, BASKETBALL AND SOCCER TO REMIND HIMSELF OF WHO HE WAS AND SO THAT HE COULD VISUALIZE HIMSELF HEALTHY

- [ ] WALK IN THE POSITIVE OUTCOME OF YOUR CHILD AS A POWERFUL SPIRIT

- [ ] COMMUNICATE WITH YOUR SON OR DAUGHTER AS A HEALTHY CHILD WITH DAILY AFFIRMATIONS

- [ ] TALK WITH HIM/HER IN A POSITIVE WAY

- [ ] TELL HIM/HER HOW SUCCESSFUL THEY WILL BE WHEN THEY GROW UP

- [ ] SHARE WITH HIM/HER HOW BEAUTIFUL AND HEALTHY THEY ARE

- [ ] IT'S OK TO SPOIL THEM, BUT DO NOT PITY THEM

- [ ] SURPRISE THEM WITH A HOME-COOKED MEAL

- [ ] START A SCRAPBOOK YOU CAN BUILD TOGETHER

What Rejuvenates You as a Parent?

It's very important to rejuvenate yourself through this adjustment. Keep yourself healthy with the right mindset.

I, myself, was exercising everyday at the hospital with a spin class and volunteering to help with animals. All of this was in an effort to rejuvenate myself, so when I walked into my son's room I could share what good things I did today. It's very important to fuel yourself and to walk in Faith with conviction of the outcome you want to achieve that day. It's important to keep yourself healthy while you're going through this adjustment, so you can be there for your son or daughter. I'm not saying it's easy. I remember going to the Faith Hill and Tim McGraw concert with a friend at Key Arena down the street from Children's hospital. The opening song was, "Live Like You Were Dying." Right then I broke down crying. But, after the concert, I was so pumped up I came right back to my son's room sharing how great the concert was. I remember how important it was for him to see me smile.

Think how you can pump yourself up to fight for your son or daughter. How can you rejuvenate yourself? What makes you happy?

☐ TAKING WALKS

☐ ATTENDING CONCERTS

☐ GOING TO THE ZOO

☐ VOLUNTEERING TO HELP

☐ GARDENING

☐ GOING TO THE GYM OR DOING YOGA, PILATES, TAI CHI OR A SPIN CLASS

☐ PAINTING

☐ HORSEBACK RIDING

☐ ATTENDING SPORTS EVENTS

☐ PRAY/MEDITATE/CHANT

REJUVENATE YOURSELF TO STAY HEALTHY

WHAT REJUVENATES YOU?

☐ _____

☐ _____

☐ _____

☐ _____

☐ _____

☐ _____

☐ _____

☐ _____

☐ _____

☐ _____

☐ _____

☐ _____

☐ _____

☐ _____

☐ _____

Reme

The i
is no
I a

mber:

lness

t who

m®

VIS UAL IZE

VISUALIZE YOUR SON OR DAUGHTER HEALTHY.

WALK IN THE OUTCOME OF YOUR SON OR DAUGHTER LEAVING THE HOSPITAL

SPEAK WELLNESS UPON YOUR CHILD

ALWAYS TALK ABOUT YOUR CHILD'S FUTURE

MAKE A STAND FOR WHO YOU ARE

BELIEVE IN WHAT YOU STAND FOR

AND STAND FOR WHAT YOU BELIEVE IN

ACTI
YO
MINI

VATE
UR
OSET

ACTIVATIONS FOR YOUR SON OR DAUGHTER:
WHATEVER YOU THINK, YOU WILL CREATE

- [ ] THINK AND WALK IN WELLNESS AND HEALTH

- [ ] THE ILLNESS YOU HAVE IS JUST A SITUATION

- [ ] THE ILLNESS IS NOT WHO YOU ARE; YOU ARE A POWERFUL SPIRIT

- [ ] YOUR GOALS AND DREAMS DON'T STOP BECAUSE OF YOUR SITUATION

- [ ] REMIND YOURSELF THAT YOU ARE NOT THE ILLNESS

- [ ] THINK OF YOURSELF AS HEALTHY

- [ ] ENVISION HOW YOU WILL LOOK AND FEEL AFTER LEAVING THE HOSPITAL

HELP YOUR SON OR DAUGHTER RECORD THEIR GOALS AND DREAMS:

☐ WHERE WILL YOU TRAVEL IN THE WORLD?

☐ WHAT WILL YOU BE WHEN YOU GROW UP?

☐ WILL YOU BE MARRIED? HAVE KIDS? HOW MANY?

☐ WHAT WILL YOU STUDY IN SCHOOL? WHERE WILL YOU GO TO COLLEGE?

☐ HOW WILL YOU CHANGE THE WORLD?

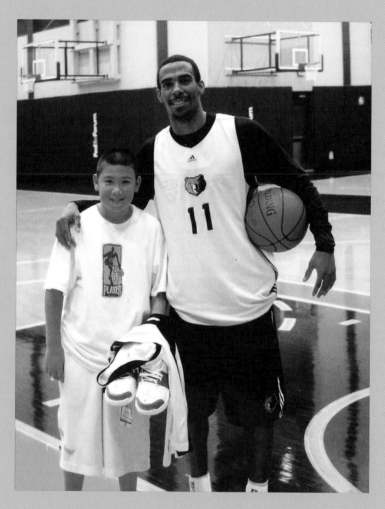

Brandon with Mike Conley, Jr.
of the Memphis Grizzlies

Brandon's goals and dreams at 10 years old

Make A Wish granted his wish and flew him to Memphis, Tennessee to play basketball with NBA player Mike Conley

Brandon's Affirmations and Goals for Recovery

1. I am going to be an NBA basketball player.
2. I am going to be married one time and have 2 kids.
3. When I leave the hospital, I'm going to bring my family to Atlantis.

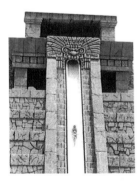 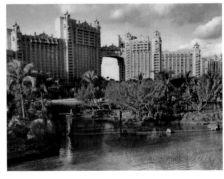

Brandon's affirmation and vision was going down the water slides at Atlantis in the Bahamas. This is Brandon 8 months later.

Brothers

- ☐ BE SUPPORTIVE AND ENGAGE WITH YOUR BROTHER/SISTER THROUGH THIS TRANSITION

- ☐ SHARE WITH YOUR BROTHER/SISTER EVERYTHING THAT IS GOING ON WITH YOUR LIFE

- ☐ SUPPORT YOUR BROTHER/SISTER AND FAMILY THROUGH THIS ADJUSTMENT

- ☐ ALWAYS WALK IN THE POSITIVE OUTCOME AND NOT NEGATIVITY

- ☐ VISIT YOUR BROTHER/SISTER AND BE WITH THEM AS MUCH AS POSSIBLE

& Sisters

- ☐ WHATEVER ACTIVITIES YOU ENGAGED IN WITH YOUR BROTHER/SISTER BEFORE THE ILLNESS, KEEP DOING THEM TO YOUR BEST ABILITY

- ☐ PLAY GAMES

- ☐ WATCH FUNNY MOVIES/FUNNY TV SHOWS

- ☐ TEXT THEM

- ☐ SKYPE WITH THEM

FAMILY MEMBERS OF THE PATIENT

1. LIVE IN THE JOY OF THE DAY (EACH DAY) BY ONLY SEEING YOUR SON OR DAUGHTER FOR THE POSSIBILITY OF WHO THEY SAY THEY ARE AND NOT THE ILLNESS

2. TREAT YOUR CHILD IN THE OUTCOME OF WELLNESS

3. ALWAYS WALK IN THE POSITIVE OUTCOME

4. START A ROTATION PLAN FOR PEOPLE TO VISIT

5. SEND PROGRESS UPDATES ON HOW YOUR SON OR DAUGHTER IS DOING, TO FAMILY, FRIENDS, AND COMMUNITY MEMBERS

GRANDPARENTS

Talk and play with your grandchild in the same way as though they are visiting your home.

Examples from Brandon's Grandparents:

☐ **PLAYING CATCH IN THE HALLWAY**

☐ **WATCHING SPORTS ON TV**

☐ **ENCOURAGING LAUGHTER**

☐ **SHOOTING BASKETS IN HIS ROOM (BRANDON HAD A BASKETBALL HOOP IN HIS ROOM)**

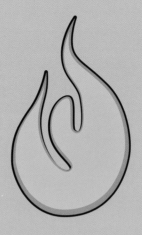

Learning the
Language of
Miracles®

REMEMBER: THE ILLNESS
IS NOT WHO I AM®

Know: You are an inspiration!

Your walk inspires others!

It takes pure courage to walk your walk!

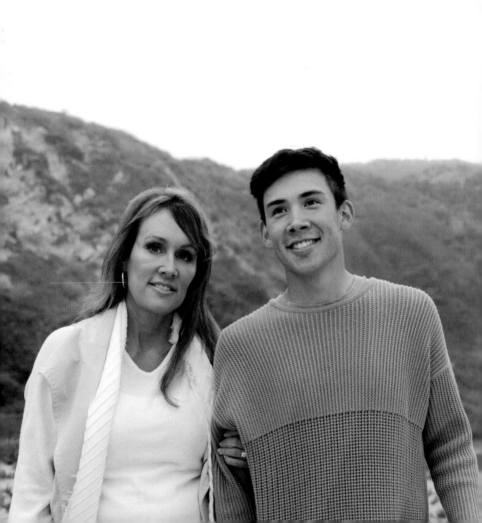

Fight and rebuke the illness

Make a stand for who you are

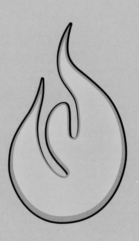

REMEMBER: THE ILLNESS IS NOT WHO I AM®

It takes
suppor
recove
ch

a village
ting the
ry of a
ld.

Friends & Community

Support from friends and the community is immeasurable — a huge impact for your son or daughter.

The greater the effort visiting, the easier the adjustment is for your child. Bring to the hospital things you would normally do at home.

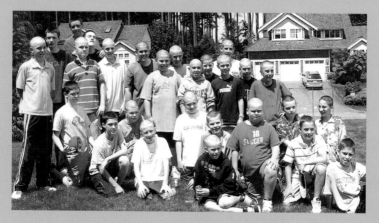

Friends of Brandon shaved their heads to support him.

- ☐ FRIENDS AND COMMUNITY MEMBERS BROUGHT MOVIES, BOARD GAMES, CARDS.

- ☐ COMMUNITY MEMBERS BROUGHT HOMEMADE MEALS AND TREATS TO THE HOSPITAL

- ☐ THEY MADE A BANNER THAT SAID "BRANDON ROCKS" WITH OVER A HUNDRED CLASSMATES' AND FRIENDS' SIGNATURES

- ☐ THEY EMBROIDERED BLANKETS AND PILLOWS

- ☐ CLASSMATES CUT THEIR HAIR IN SOLIDARITY AS THEY DIDN'T WANT BRANDON TO FEEL ALONE. IT PUT THEM IN THE SAME PLACE WITH BRANDON.

Teachers

- ☐ MAKE AN EFFORT TO STAY IN COMMUNICATION AS MUCH AS POSSIBLE WITH THE STUDENT

- ☐ DO NOT TREAT THEM DIFFERENTLY JUST BECAUSE THEY HAVE AN ILLNESS

- ☐ YOU MAY HAVE TO DO SIMPLER LESSONS, BUT NEVER MAKE THE CHILD FEEL LIKE THEY ARE BEHIND

- ☐ INSTEAD, FOCUS ON BEING PRESENT IN WHAT THE CHILD IS DOING THAT DAY

- ☐ TRY TO KEEP THE CHILD UP TO DATE WITH NOT ONLY CLASS MATERIAL BUT WHAT IS GOING ON

- ☐ AT THE SCHOOL AS A WHOLE AND WHAT THEY HAVE TO LOOK FORWARD TO

- ☐ TELL THEM ABOUT SCHOOL ASSEMBLIES, SCHOOL SPORTS TEAMS, CLUBS, CHANGES TO THE SCHOOL, THINGS THAT HAPPEN WITH THEIR PEERS OR OTHER TEACHERS OR STAFF (MAYBE THERE'S A NEW LUNCH BEING SERVED THEY CAN LOOK FORWARD TO)

COACHES

☐ **MAKE AN EFFORT TO STAY IN COMMUNICATION AS MUCH AS POSSIBLE WITH THE CHILD YOU COACH**

☐ **KEEP THEM UP TO SPEED ON EVERYTHING THAT'S GOING ON WITH THE TEAM**

☐ **WHEN YOU VISIT, TAKE PLAY BOOKS AND VIDEOS OF PRACTICES OR GAMES TO SHOW THEM**

My son and I are here to
help you with your fight.

This is the fight of your life

We believe in you

Your gifts are inside of you

This was our fight and
Brandon and I are here to
share our Gifts, because
we know you have the
same gifts within you.

THE ILLNESS IS NOT WHO
YOU ARE®

BRANDON'S MIRACLE

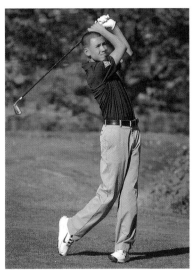

BRANDON 8 YEARS LATER ON THE
WOODINVILLE HIGH SCHOOL GOLF TEAM

Brandon did not allow his illness to affect his goals and dreams he had for the future. He proved to be a powerful being and a cancer survivor.

Today, my son is cancer free. This would never have been possible without the help and support from members of our whole community. I am here today to share Brandon's story and share with people how influential Speaking the Language of Miracles can be for a child or loved one dealing with an illness.

BRANDON
TODAY...

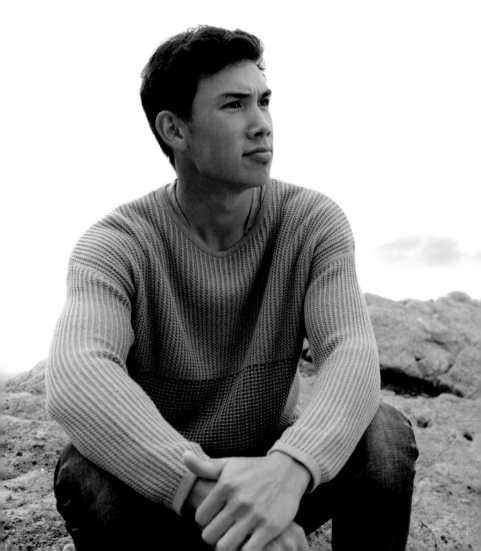

Brandon in his own words:
I am very thankful for Children's Hospital.

I have been cancer-free for more than 11 years. I have God, my mother, Deanna Scott, my sister, Taylor, and my family to thank for this incredible blessing; and because the illness was never, ever who I was. I chose to not live in the situation.

I remember thinking: I can create anything I put my mind to. If you believe it and you're passionate about it, you can accomplish it. There's so much negative energy in the world. I know it's really hard to make changes. We are creatures of habit; some good and some bad. We all have bad days and it's easy to dwell on bad breaks, but as soon as you learn to let go and tackle these unfortunate events with a single statement: The situation is not who I am, you will feel powerful and free to live the life you want to live.

Just by taking a step back and saying, "Okay, this situation isn't who I am, it doesn't define me. What can I change? How can I learn and better myself?" I believe there's always a positive in every situation you encounter and there is room to grow and become a better person.

With this book, it can help people live a healthier, happier life. Knowing they can make a positive impact in their own lives and on others around them, just by being a positive contribution. What this book will do for anyone who reads it… is truly amazing. I hope you remember who you really are and this book will offer clarity to see all the gifts inside.

I believe everyone should read this book. It will unlock so many doors, you never thought possible. I want people to unlock the gifts within themselves. This book will empower you to make a difference in your own lives and in the world; giving you confidence to create the life you love.

A final message to Seattle Children's Hospital

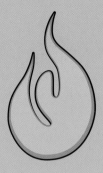

My reason for sharing Speaking the Language of Miracles is to give back to Children's Hospital what they gave back to me— **my son, Brandon.**

TWENTY PERCENT (20%) OF THE NET PROCEEDS FROM BOOK SALES GOES DIRECTLY TO SUPPORT CHILDREN'S HOSPITALS.

CHAPTER

02

Lifestyle

CREATE THE LIFE YOU LOVE

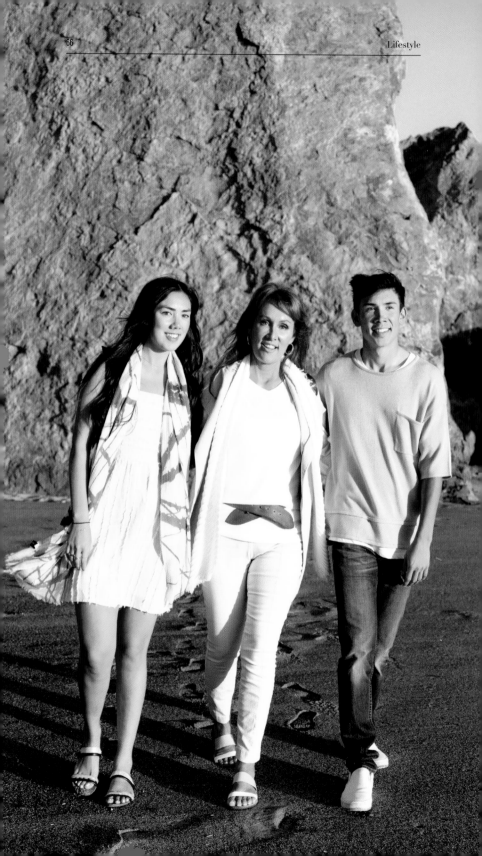

How to Apply Speaking the Language of Miracles® to Your Life

Speaking the Language of Miracles ignites the flame within you. The flame represents God's spirit. My belief is that everyone has God's spirit within him or herself. Our language is the most powerful gift that we have. With our word, we can create a beautiful life.

1. Ask yourself: Is your heart open to the gifts that are inside of you? Watch the miracle take place.
2. With Speaking the Language of Miracles, you can make the distinctions if you are using your gifts.
3. Teach Speaking the Language of Miracles to family, friends, community members and whomever you encounter.
4. Remind everyone that the situation they are dealing with or encounter does not change who they are as an individual. Walk in the positive outcome of who you are.

THE TIME IS NOW

REMEMBER: WHEN YOU ARE PRESENT

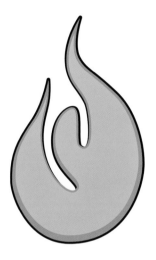

YOU ARE THE MOST POWERFUL WHEN YOU ARE IN THE NOW

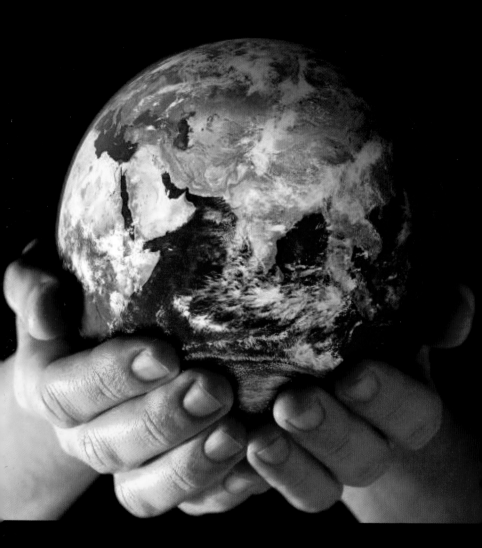

Kids are our Future

Each and every one of us makes a ripple effect in the world. What's the ripple effect that you want to create?

DREAI

YOU

THE W

M BIG.
ARE
ORLD.

DREAM BIG
Anything you think you will create

WHAT WILL YOU BE WHEN YOU GROW UP?

_____

_____

_____

WHAT DO YOU HAVE ENVISIONED FOR YOUR FUTURE?

_____

_____

_____

HOW WILL YOU CHANGE THE WORLD?

_____

_____

_____

HOW WILL YOU MAKE THE WORLD A BETTER PLACE?

_____

_____

_____

Everything that we were taught and everything that was instilled in us when we were little, is what we use today. Some of us have been derailed because of our situations, and have created stories that we hide behind. I truly want you to know how beautiful you are. And, what is inside of you is much more powerful than any situation. God created you Perfect and Beautiful in every way.

REMEMBER,
THE SITUATION IS NOT WHO YOU ARE.®

Surround yourself with positive people and watch your Dreams become a reality.

Situations

ALWAYS MAKE DISTINCTIONS OF WHAT THE SITUATION IS:

Media, Bad News, Drama, Gossip, Divorce, Death, Illness, Jealousy, Hate, He said-She said, Liar liar pants on fire. Situations are always negative, they rob us of who we are! We are much greater than any situation. People who create drama are joy stealers. Never partake in their situation. Instead, have empathy for that person that is going through a hard time. Remind them the situation is not who they are. Surround yourself with positive, happy, creative, successful people who Dream Big. When you hang out with successful people, it's contagious.

THE POSITIVE THINGS WE SAY ARE WHAT WE ATTRACT BACK TO US.

Listen to the words you are saying, are they positive or negative? The situation is the enemy in many forms. The enemy wants you to walk in the situation. The enemy wants you to be powerless. The enemy wants you to walk in sickness, broken relationships, failing businesses and recessions. The enemy does not want you to walk in solutions. The enemy does not want you to walk in the outcome of success. The enemy does not want you to walk in your God-given gifts. The enemy will always want us to stay in the situation. But we are victorious and we will conquer the situation.

If you have identified that you are always sharing negative situations, the good news is: it's not who you are. You can have the clarity to make the choice to change that mindset. And, guess how long it takes to make that change?...

IN AN INSTANT!

Your la
can c
your li
ins

nguage

hange

e in an

ant

WHAT IS YOUR WORLD VISION?

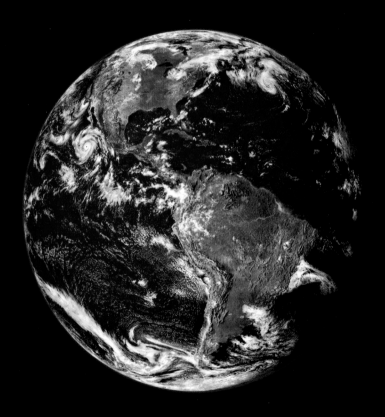

CREATE WORLD PEACE WITH SPEAKING THE LANGUAGE OF MIRACLES.

THE SITUATION IS OUR ENEMY. NOT EACH OTHER.

ALL IT TAKES IS A MINDSET TO HAVE WORLD PEACE.

MAKE THE DISTINCTION THAT THE SITUATION IS OUR ENEMY AND NOT EACH OTHER.

I "CHOOSE" TO BE PRO-HUMANITY. NO MORE WARS. ALL IT TAKES IS ONE PERSON, ONE VOICE TO UNITE US.

WHAT IS THE OUTCOME OF NO MORE WARS?

INSTEAD OF SPENDING TRILLIONS OF DOLLARS TO DESTROY OUR PLANET AND EACH OTHER, WE CAN TAKE THAT MONEY AND SAVE OUR PLANET AND CREATE A BETTER WORLD.

WE HAVE THE POWER, TECHNOLOGY AND LANGUAGE TO CREATE A BETTER WORLD.

WALK HERE ON EARTH AS YOU WOULD IN HEAVEN.

CREATE YOUR WORLD AS IF IT WAS IN HEAVEN.

IMAGINE WHAT THE WORLD WOULD LOOK LIKE WITH WORLD PEACE.

OUR GOAL IS TO BE "ONE" WITH THE UNIVERSE, THAT "ONE" IS WALKING IN THE POWER OF NOW. THE POWER OF NOW IS GOD INSIDE OF US. GOD IS THE ONE.

LIVE YOUR LIFE.

YOU ARE THE CREATOR OF YOUR LIFE.

DAILY AFFIRMATIONS

WHEN YOU SAY YOUR I AM'S, IT'S IMPORTANT TO KNOW WHAT'S INSIDE OF YOU. YOUR I AM'S CAN'T COME FROM EGO.

YOUR I AM'S COME FROM KNOWING GOD'S SPIRIT IS INSIDE EACH AND EVERYONE OF US. WHEN YOU ARE WALKING IN SOLUTIONS, YOU ARE WALKING IN THE NOW.

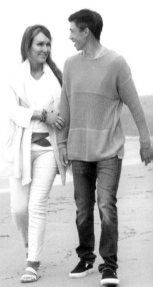

THAT'S WHEN YOU ARE WALKING IN VICTORY.

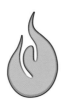

- [ ] I AM A HEALTHY CHILD OF GOD
- [ ] I AM RECEIVING ALL GREAT BLESSINGS TODAY
- [ ] I AM A POWERFUL SPIRIT
- [ ] I AM WALKING IN JOY
- [ ] I AM HAPPY
- [ ] I AM BEAUTIFUL
- [ ] I AM LOVING
- [ ] I AM GIVING
- [ ] I AM FORGIVING
- [ ] I AM CARING
- [ ] I AM SUCCESSFUL
- [ ] I AM A MAJOR CONTRIBUTION TO MY FAMILY, FRIENDS AND COMMUNITY
- [ ] I AM OF MY WORD
- [ ] I AM TRUSTING
- [ ] I AM LOYAL
- [ ] I AM A LEADER
- [ ] I AM POWERFUL
- [ ] I AM A SURVIVOR

Choices

EVERY CHOICE YOU MAKE
CAUSES A RIPPLE EFFECT
IN EVERYTHING YOU DO. NO
MATTER HOW BIG OR SMALL,
KNOW WHAT YOUR GIFTS ARE,
AND KNOW HOW POWERFUL
YOU ARE. LISTEN TO YOUR
LANGUAGE. DO YOU CHOOSE
TO MAKE YOUR CHOICES
POSITIVE OR NEGATIVE?

IT'S EASY MAKING THE
RIGHT CHOICES. WHEN YOU
LOOK AT THE OUTCOME
OF WHAT YOU WANT TO
CREATE, IS IT?...

Positive
or
Negative

YOU CAN MAKE YOUR
DREAMS COME TRUE
WITH THE RIGHT CHOICES.

Cha

your

insta

nge
ᵖ life
ɪntly

Staying Focused on **Creating Your Dreams** is Walking In The Language Of Miracles

By walking in the Language of Miracles you make choices that create opportunities for you to be successful. It's never too early and it's never too late to start making the right choices.

It's up to you to decide where you want to go and what you want to do, what choices will help you and which ones will hinder you.

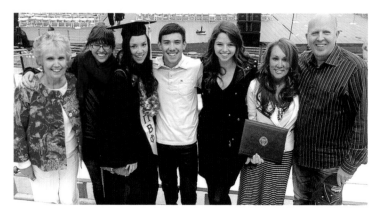

My daughter Taylor, "walked in the outcome" and graduated from the University of Washington. She then went on to land her dream job in Los Angeles to create a life she loves

TAILOR THESE CHOICES TO YOUR OWN AMBITIONS:

BEING GOAL-MINDED WORKS

FIND SOMETHING YOU LOVE TO DO:

- Focus on obtaining your dream job 5, 10 and 20 years or further down the road
- What choices will elevate you towards landing that job?

CREATE LONG-TERM GOALS

Examples:

- If you're in high school, in what industry of work do you want to be in after college?
- If you're in college, what type of boss do you want to be one day?
- If you were to be alive at the reading of your eulogy, what would you want someone to write and say about you?

IF YOU DON'T KNOW WHAT YOU LOVE TO DO YET, CREATE SHORT-TERM OBTAINABLE GOALS.

Examples:
- Landing a job interview
- Making a sports team
- Improving your academic performance
- Learning new skills

SURROUND YOURSELF WITH LEADERS

FIND MENTORS YOU LOOK UP TO FROM WHOM YOU CAN LEARN

- Teachers, counselors, colleagues, bosses, family members
- Make it a point to stay in contact with people who inspire you or to whom you look up to
  - Schedule a coffee or lunch
  - Ask them for advice, learn from the experiences of your leaders and mentors.
- If you don't have many physical mentors:
  - Find authors or speakers who you can read and listen to (TED talks, podcasts, autobiographies, community seminars)

Practice Makes Perfect

- Practice pushing yourself forward, constantly finding new opportunities, and take ahold of and follow through on them.
- Practice finding a routine that will benefit your life and your future. Ask about your mentors and successful individuals' daily routines. Fine tune what you learn from them and create your own routine.
- Practice finding as many work experiences as early as possible.
- Practice writing everything out
  – Keep a journal or write in your phone "notes" section. Write everything down (ideas that come to mind, accomplishments you envision yourself achieving)
- Practice communicating with multiple personalities and different types of people of different backgrounds
- Practice being a go-getter rather than waiting to be asked to do something
- Practice Visualizing - While saying your affirmation envision your own future outcomes.

EXAMPLES:

- Holding a college acceptance letter
  – What will you study? Where you will live on campus? How will it feel?
- Receiving a job offer
  – How will you respond? What exactly will they offer you? How will you accept?
- Delivering a presentation
  – Who will be in the room?
  – To whom will you direct your attention?
  – What do you want to get across?
  – What questions will you answer?

YOU ARE AMAZING. WALK IN THE GIFTS THAT ARE IN YOU.

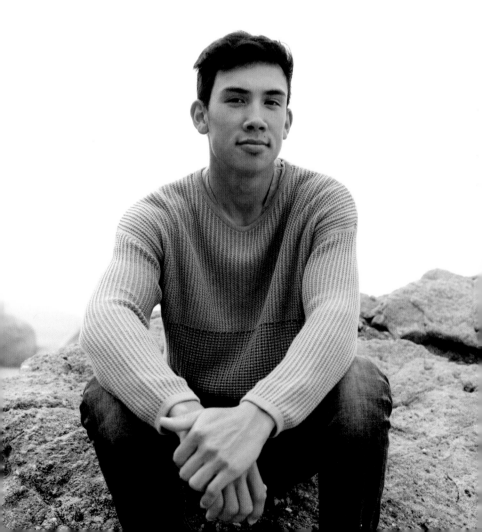

CHAPTER

03

Business

**WHATEVER YOUR MINDSET IS, IT SETS
THE FOUNDATION FOR YOUR BUSINESS SUCCESS**

Speaking The Language of Miracles® In Business

Accounting	Information Technology
Attorneys at Law	Law Enforcement
Banking	Manufacturing
CEOs	Marketing
Construction	Medicine
Customer Service	Public Safety
Education	Real Estate
Executive Management	Software Development
Government	Transportation
Human Resources	Venture Capital

...AND HUNDREDS OF OTHER FIELDS

WHAT IS SPEAKING THE LANGUAGE OF MIRACLES IN BUSINESS?

To not walk in the situation.

The situation is not who you are. Whatever you talk about, it will persist and grow. So, that is why you want to talk in and about solutions. Write out your solutions, implement and take action to your solutions. Make distinctions as to what is working in your company. Stop talking about what's not working. That is attracting negative energy back to you. It's impossible to walk in solutions when you are walking in the situation.

Stop talking about other companies, it's not greener on the other side. The green is inside of you. You are the winning formula.

When you walk in this mindset, you see your unique gifts and your talents flow out of you. You see yourself inspired. The Language of Miracles brings out your Higher Purpose.

All because you choose not to walk in the situation.

When you are walking in solutions, you are walking in the power of NOW

You are the most powerful when you are in the NOW

Wha

you t

you c

ever
hink,
reate.

To walk in the positive outcome you need to remember one thing:

THE SITUATION IS NOT WHO YOU ARE.®

All it takes is the Distinction of the right language to attract what you want in your business.

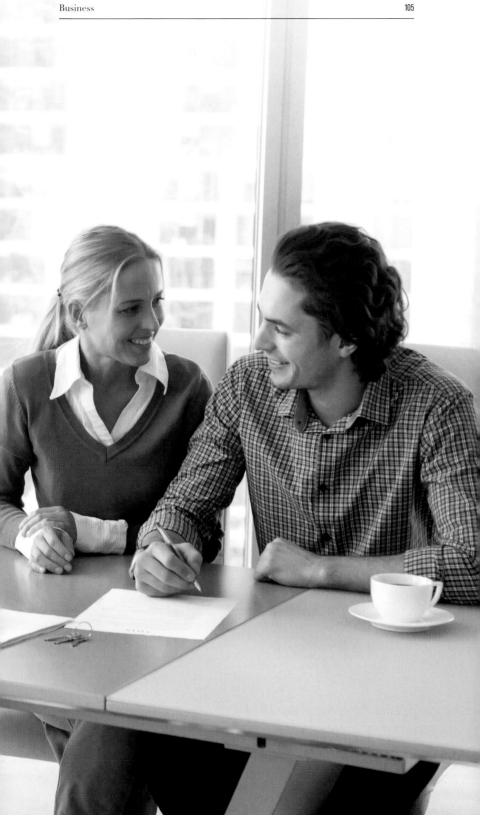

Deanna's Business Experience

In 2008, my dog grooming business was very successful. I was getting new referrals every day from existing clients who would give out my name and number. I never advertised my business. It was all by word of mouth. When my friends and other business owners would ask me how I was doing so well in this recession, I would reply back and say: **THE RECESSION IS NOT WHO I AM. IT'S JUST A SITUATION!!!** I have a mindset that my business is thriving, I walk in the outcome of what I want to achieve everyday and consistently be my very best.

The Power of My Day

Affirmations every morning help me walk in the intent of what I want to achieve this day and every day.

Before I rise in the morning, I say my affirmations:

- I am receiving all great blessings today (Doesn't that feel good? Starts my day off great!)
- I am a contribution to my clients
- I love my work
- I love my clients
- I am walking in financial abundance
- I have new clients every day
- I am successful
- I am the greatest
- I am happy

AND BECAUSE I MADE A CHOICE TO BEGIN MY DAY WITH SUCH A GREAT START, I RECEIVE ALL GREAT BLESSINGS THROUGHOUT THE DAY. I WALK IN THE INTENT OF MY AFFIRMATIONS. I GIVE MY THANKS TO GOD TO BE MY VERY BEST. I THANK GOD THROUGHOUT MY DAY, AND I AM VERY GRATEFUL AND THANKFUL FOR THE CLIENTS I HAVE.

DISTINCTIONS

My paradise is in front of me every day. It's just that I have the clarity to see I'm creating it.

And now so do you, all it takes is:

CLARITY = Making distinctions.

CHOICES = Positive or negative? When you look at the outcome of what you want to achieve, ask yourself if it's positive or negative – it's easy to make the right choices. Focus on the Positive Outcome.

ACCOUNTABILITY = Own your life. Own your mistakes. Do not blame others.

INTEGRITY = Trust; be someone of your word. Without your word, you're nothing. Follow up with what you say.

Look at the outcome of following up with your word, and then look at the outcome of NOT following up with your word. To be successful in business you need to trust the person you're doing business with.

Your language is everything. When you follow up with your word, people can trust you.

YOU

...are the winning formula

YOUR MINDSET IS A CHOICE

This Is How to Have a Healthier Mindset Within Your Business

Write down the situation and put it up on the wall, step back, and watch yourself get inspired.

THE SITUATION IS NOT WHO YOU ARE.

Walk & Talk in Solutions

- Make Distinctions
- Reinvent
- What is the outcome you want?
- Take Action
- Implement
- Have a Positive Mindset

Choices *and* Distinctions

You are the Winning Formula

So often we choose to walk in the situation and when we do, we don't see who we are and what we are capable of. The situation robs us of our God-given unique gifts of who we are.

You are much more Powerful than any Situation.

Choose to apply your gifts that are inside of you, to walk and talk in Solutions. Your gifts overcome any situation. All you need is the mindset to choose to walk in solutions

WHATEVER YOUR MINDSET IS, IT SETS THE FOUNDATION FOR YOUR BUSINESS' SUCCESS.

WE ALL HAVE FREE WILL TO MAKE THE CHOICES IN OUR LIVES.

Whatever you think, you will create. Have you ever been inspired by someone and said, "I wish I could do that" or "I wish I could make as much as that person", but make excuses why you can't? It's because these individuals love what they are doing. Make the right choice — are you in the right job or career?

Just know there isn't anything you can't have today. What is your self talk? The only thing stopping you is yourself. If there's anything you don't like in your life, you need to look in the mirror. You have attracted everything that you have today: good and bad . . . hopefully more good.

What I'm trying to identify with you is that all the good things you have in your life today are from a positive mindset that is inside of you. You didn't achieve these great things in your life with a negative mindset. My wish for you is to quadruple your positive mindset and create a life that you love. My goal is to remind you of who you are. You are victorious.

YOU ARE THE CREATOR OF YOUR LIFE, DREAM BIG!

WHAT DO YOU WANT TO ACCOMPLISH?

WHAT ARE THE OUTCOMES?

DESCRIBE YOUR OUTCOMES

- [ ]
- [ ]
- [ ]
- [ ]
- [ ]
- [ ]
- [ ]
- [ ]
- [ ]
- [ ]
- [ ]
- [ ]
- [ ]
- [ ]
- [ ]
- [ ]
- [ ]

WHO ARE YOU IN MEETINGS?

- **Office Meetings**
- **Leadership Meetings**
- **Strategy Meetings**
- **Board Meetings**

When you're in your group meetings, do you leave just talking about the problems and situations, or do you leave feeling inspired, energized; walking and talking in Solutions?

WHAT ARE YOUR SOLUTIONS?

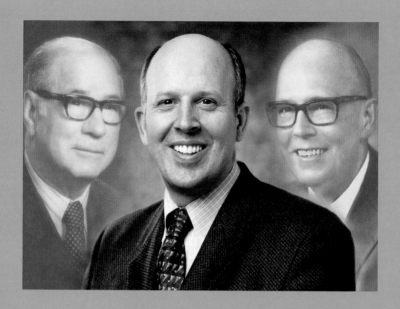

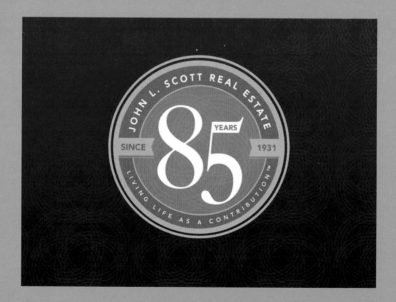

John L. Scott®
REAL ESTATE

Real Estate Testimonial

APPLYING SPEAKING THE LANGUAGE OF MIRACLES IN BUSINESS AT JOHN L. SCOTT REAL ESTATE

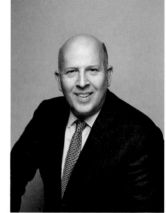

Chairman and CEO:
J. Lennox Scott

J. Lennox Scott is a third generation Chairman and CEO of John L. Scott Real Estate, which was founded by his grandfather in Seattle in 1931. From the beginning, John L. Scott's success has been from its focus on each individual client.

Lennox is consistently recognized as one of the Top 10 Megabrokers in the nation.

Lennox is highly involved with the National Association of Realtors, Real Estate Services Advisory Group.

John L. Scott has over 110 offices with more than 3,000 sales associates in the states of Washington, Oregon, Idaho and California.

John L. Scott closes over 35,000 transactions for over 12 billion dollars in sales volume on an annual basis.

When I met Deanna on December 13, 2008, I could tell instantly that she was a powerful spirit. A few weeks after meeting her, I had the opportunity to ask her how she was so successful during the economic collapse that our country was going through at that time... That's when she said "the recession is not who I am." Deanna shared she does not listen to the news media or negative talk; "I only walk in the outcome of what I want to achieve." her speaking resonated with me. It psychologically and emotionally took me to a higher state of being.

WHAT INSPIRED ME WAS DEANNA'S STATEMENT:

THE SITUATION IS NOT WHO YOU ARE.

The Great Recession

In the year 2007, the housing market started to deteriorate. Then in year 2008, it accelerated downward to substantially lower sales activity and prices. It would have been easy to make the statement that this is a terrible housing market and then just wallow in it.

I have always been a positive person, but then I met Deanna and she helped elevate my spirit through her approach in creating distinctions and, more importantly, being relentlessly focused on the positive outcome.

DISTINCTION:
"The recession is not who I am"

POSITIVE OUTCOME:
"I am successful, I am a major contribution to my clients, I am Walking in Abundance."

Positive Mind Set is at the core of success. It's who you are. Your higher purpose is helping your clients.

Your mindset psychologically is the inspiration that helps you create personal motivation to move forward to accomplish, to provide a higher level of service, and to walk in joy within your work.

Today, we are excelling to greater heights with Speaking the Language of Miracles but there always seems to be a recession every ten years. Although the next one will be shorter in duration than the Great Recession, we are already prepared for the situation. We will walk in success. We will walk in the positive outcome.

CURRENT EXAMPLE: SHORTAGE OF INVENTORY OF HOMES FOR SALE.

Instead of accepting this as fact and placing yourself as a victim, what are you going to do about it?

That's where positive affirmations come into play.

"I find Homeowners who *want* to sell their home."

This is what I state each day on the way to work. So, by the time I get into the office I am in action.

Instead of dwelling in the situation, walk in the outcome of what you want to achieve.

Write up the situation in a few words, print it on a piece of paper and tape it to a wall; step back and take a look. Then the next important step:

What are you going to do about it?

What is the positive outcome that you want?

Focus on solutions to handle and overcome the situation, then detail out your action steps to accomplish this.

Personal Business Affirmations

- I am a Powerful Spirit
- I am a major contribution to my Clients
- I am walking in abundance in my Career
- I am Financially Successful
- I am walking in the Positive Outcome

THINK BIG – DREAM BIGGER

Fully express yourself; continually go through a renewal of spirit.

We have always done Strategic Planning and Business Plans at work which is a form of Thinking Big. But Speaking the Language of Miracles has brought it alive and keeps our momentum moving forward by making declarations of your service and personal commitments.

When I first met Deanna, after hearing her language and concepts, I made the statement:

"I can see I'm not thinking big enough"

WE HAVE BEEN APPLYING SPEAKING THE LANGUAGE OF MIRACLES TO WALK IN SUCCESS IN EVERYTHING WE DO

THINK BIG. DREAM BIGGER.

Make Distinctions

It's easy making the right choices when you look at the outcome that you want to achieve.

Make distinctions, is it *Positive* or *Negative*?

What didn't work? Move forward.

Make distinctions. What is working?

Have the clarity to know when you're walking and talking in the situation...
THAT'S DEFEAT.

Nothing can change when you're walking and talking in the situation. Have the clarity to know that it's a negative. We don't have the time to walk in the situation. This is the Internet world. Everything happens in an instant. Speaking the Language of Miracles is the fastest way out of the situation. Greatness is in our DNA.

Distinctions within Real Estate

When you say there is a shortage of homes for sale to a co-worker or client, what are you attracting back to you? What's the outcome?

Instead

When you say this is a great time to buy and sell to a co-worker, client, and everyone else — what are you attracting back to you?

What's the outcome to this mindset?

All it takes is a mind shift to have the clarity to use your language to attract what you want.

It takes *courage* to walk in solutions

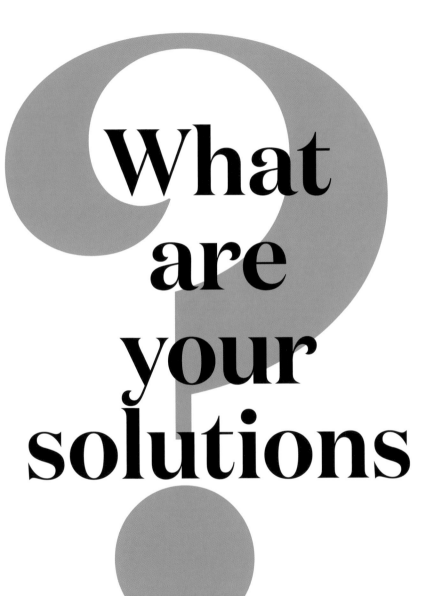

What are your solutions

EVERY MORNING WALK IN YOUR SUCCESS. EVERY DAY WALK IN THE OUTCOME.

EVERY EVENING, REMEMBER YOUR STEPS TOWARDS SUCCESS.

You are the winning formula.

Speaking the Language of Miracles® is the winning formula.

04

Sports

EVERY PLAY IS A NEW BEGINNING

Speaking The Language of Miracles® In Sports

Archery	Golf
Baseball	Hockey
Basketball	Nascar
Bowling	Sailing
Equestrian Sports	Soccer
Fencing	Softball
Football	Track & Field
Formula One Racing	Volleyball

...AND HUNDREDS MORE

"I AM THE GREATEST."

– MUHAMMED ALI

Every practice is an opportunity,

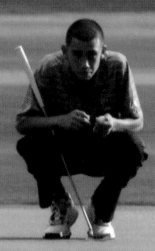

an opportunity to <u>own</u> your game.

Have a mental image of the outcome to every play.

Actions for achievement

Watch videos of yourself in action to see if your mind and body are in alignment with what you want to achieve.

WRITE OUT AFFIRMATIONS SPECIFIC TO YOU AND DECLARE YOUR LIST OUT LOUD EVERYDAY WHEN YOU GET OUT OF BED, BEFORE A GAME, WITH YOUR TEAM, AND ANYWHERE ELSE YOU CAN.

EXAMPLES:
I AM THE GREATEST FOOTBALL, BASEBALL, GOLF, BASKETBALL, HOCKEY, SOCCER, HORSEBACK, RUGBY, ETC.... PLAYER OR PERFORMER.

Visu
your
winn

alize
rself
ning.

CHAPTER

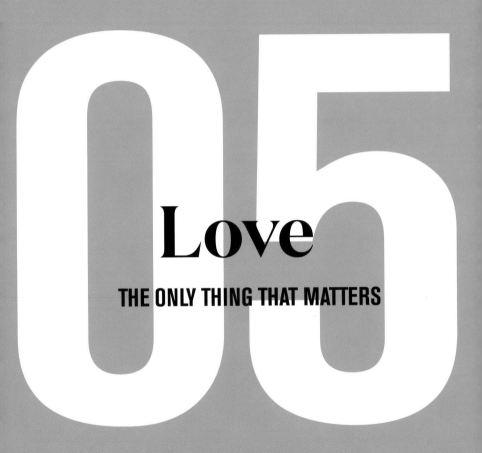

Love

THE ONLY THING THAT MATTERS

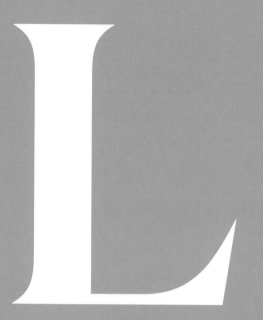

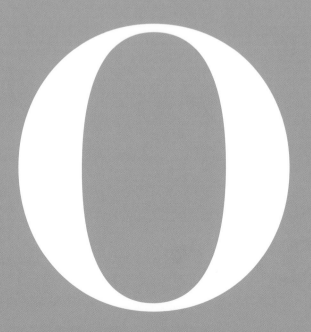

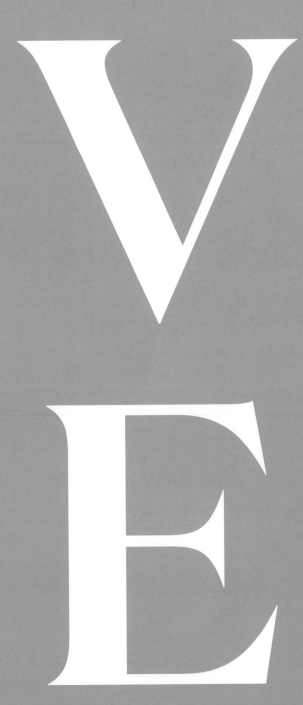

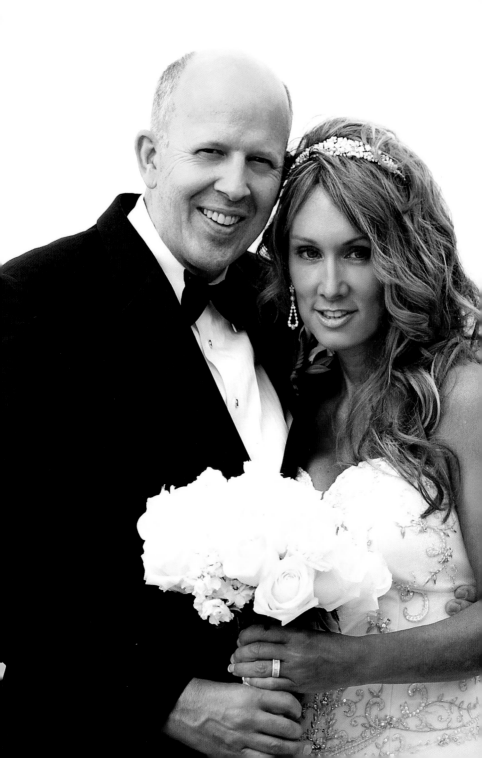

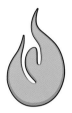

Learn How to use The Language of Miracles® in Relationships & Marriage

MARI

RIAGE

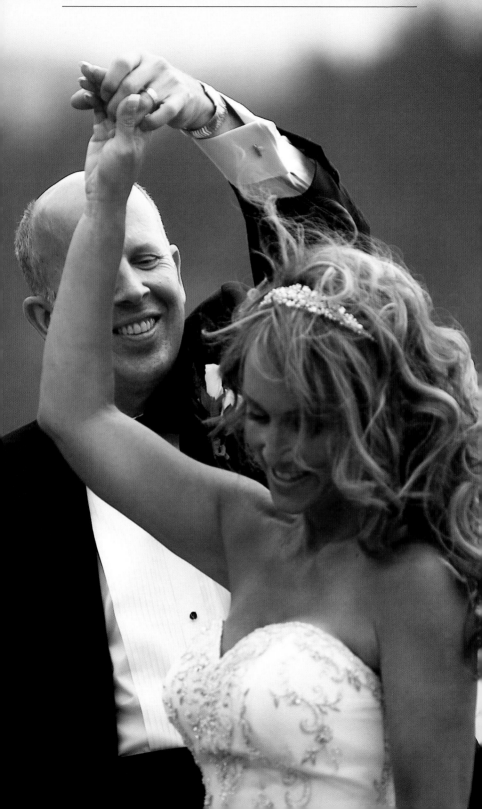

Marriage

My husband, Lennox and I, both walk in success by Speaking the Language of Miracles in every aspect of our lives. We put God first in everything we do and continuously walk in the outcome.

We reinvent ourselves through our marriage, our children, business, and our goals & dreams by making distinctions. This means that when certain situations arise, good or bad, we separate them from who we are as individuals. We say to ourselves, "That is not who I am, it is just a situation." By taking this approach, we are able to walk in who we are and not in the situation.

We say our affirmation every morning before getting out of bed. We walk in love every day with each other and give thanks for all our blessings. When we complete one goal or dream, we make new ones because whatever you think and declare, you will create. So dream big and think positive because your best days are ahead of you. All it takes is a mindset for you to live and create a life you love.

When situations occur, we make the distinctions of what the situation is and walk in our desired outcome. By doing so you can walk in success within your business, relationships, wellness and your overall life. You cannot change things if you are walking in the situation.

Instead, you can see change take place by taking yourself out of the situation and, by doing so, great things will happen!

You a
cree
of you

re the
ator
r life.

YOU ARE THE CREATOR OF YOUR LIFE

Whatever you think you will Create

You cannot have a future if you are living in past pain, whether in Relationships, Business or Life.

I'm reminding you, you are the creator of your life. What is in your DNA is much greater than any situation. Picture yourself on a white canvas. What will you create? Don't allow the situation on your canvas! It makes it impossible to move forward in life. Our situations do not serve us; we must let them go! And only keep the joy, laughter, and love on our canvas. What does your canvas look like? And we must always remember:

THE SITUATION IS NOT WHO WE ARE!

Remember, with our word we can create a beautiful life OR with our word we can destroy everything around us. You are meant to have abundance in every part of your life. The only thing stopping you is yourself. Whatever you think, you will create.

SO DREAM BIG AND THINK POSITIVE!

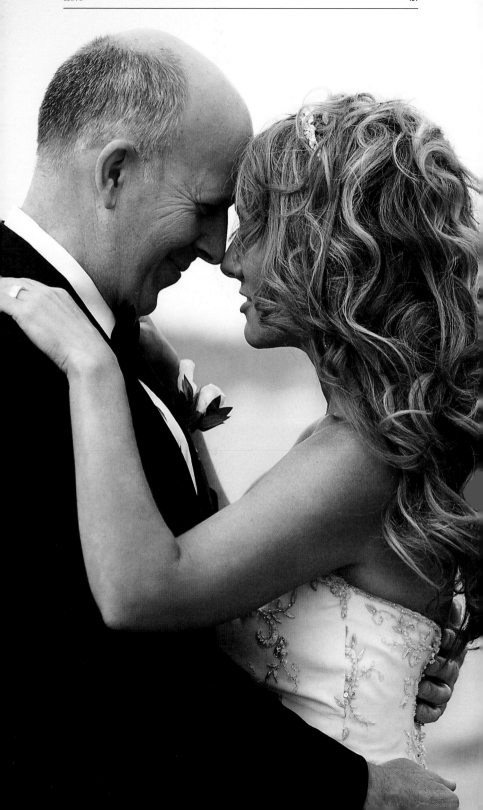

CHAPTER

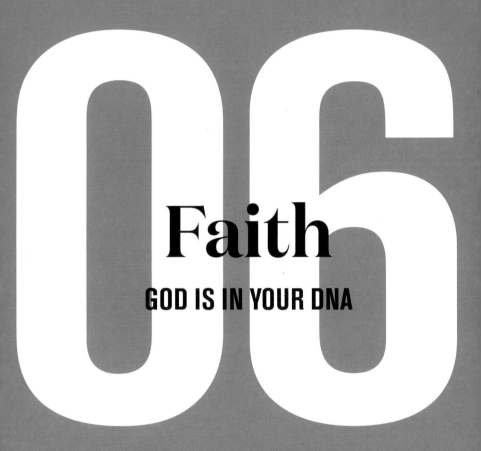

Faith

GOD IS IN YOUR DNA

WITHIN YOUR OWN INDIVIDUAL FAITH, IT'S IMPORTANT TO SPEAK WITH CONVICTION OF THE OUTCOME YOU WANT TO ACHIEVE.

YOU ARE AMAZING

Encourage every Faith

Your word is the most
powerful gift we have.
Your word is a Gift that
comes directly from God.
It is through your word you
manifest everything.
With our word we can create
a beautiful life or with
our word we can destroy
everything around us.

Bel
in wha
pray

eve
at you
y for

FAITH

Brandon would pray as if his prayers were already answered.

THANK YOU GOD, IN THE NAME OF JESUS, I AM A HEALTHY CHILD OF GOD.

THANK YOU GOD, IN THE NAME OF JESUS, I AM RECEIVING ALL GREAT BLESSINGS TODAY.

THANK YOU GOD, IN THE NAME OF JESUS, I HAVE HEALTHY BLOOD CELLS THROUGHOUT MY ENTIRE BODY.

We turned everything over to God and saw miracles every day.

Thank You, God

Thank You, Jesus

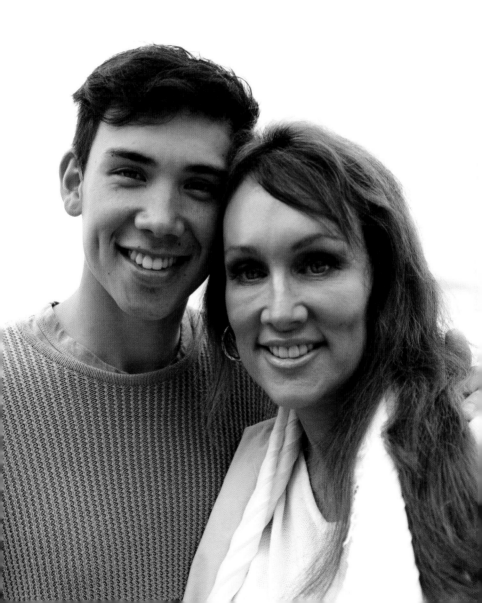

Encouragement of Faith

What is faith? The best description comes from the Bible - the resource for building faith.

"Faith is the confidence that we hope for will actually happen; it gives us assurance about the things we cannot see." - Hebrews 11:1

"I tell you the truth, if you have faith even as small as a mustard seed, you could say to this mountain, 'Move from here to there,' and it would move. Nothing would be impossible." - Matthew 17:20

There are times when our faith comes under incredible seasons of testing. Maybe you have found yourself wrestling with doubt, fear and unbelief in a circumstance beyond your control. It's critical that at these times, when you are at your weakest and most faithless point, that you be mindful of what you say because your words are like seeds. Once spoken out into the world, in time your words will bring a harvest. So speak your desired outcome and declare that your dreams for the future will come to reality, no matter what you see around you.

Are you wrestling with a situation that is challenging your faith on every side?

What is your dream? What is the "Mountain" standing in your way?

Speaking the Language of Miracles is here to help you through this time in your life, to help you take hold of your God-given promises. Believe and declare your dreams come true. Here are some declarations that will help you get started (and feel free to personalize these statements by inserting your name or loved one's name wherever it is appropriate).

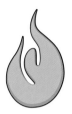

- ☐ **THE ILLNESS IS NOT WHO YOU ARE AND IT IS TRESPASSING ON GOD'S PROPERTY! (YOU!)**

- ☐ **I AM NOT WHO PEOPLE SAY I AM (SICK, POOR, DYING, UNABLE, ETC.) I AM WHO GOD SAYS I AM.**

- ☐ **GOD SAYS I AM MORE THAN VICTORIOUS THROUGH HIM WHO LOVES ME.**

- ☐ **GOD SAYS THAT GREATER IS HE THAT IS IN ME.**

forgiveness

To forgive, to be grateful, and to extend gratitude are very important parts of your life. You can watch your life transform with forgiveness & gratefulness, with the expression of gratitude.

Make distinctions regarding the "outcome" of forgiveness and then make the distinctions regarding "not" forgiving. What is the outcome?

Forgiveness does not mean having to continue to put yourself in that place of hurt. Forgiveness is a part of going forward so you do not remain hurt. You cannot have a future if you are living in past pain.

grat

itude

WRITE OUT AND DECLARE OUT LOUD EVERY DAY WHAT YOU ARE THANKFUL FOR

GOD SAYS I AM VICTORIOUS THROUGH HIM WHO LOVES ME

WALK IN THE OUTCOME WITH GOD.

YOU CAN APPLY THIS MINDSET IN EVERY PART OF YOUR LIFE TO WALK IN A BETTER OUTCOME.

WALK IN THE GIFTS THAT ARE IN YOU.

Life Transitions

How to Apply Speaking Language of Miracles to Your Life Transitions

Speaking the Language of Miracles helps you walk in the spirit of who you are.

All the love, energy and gifts that are inside of you – you take with you to your next life.

Distinctions

Imagine walking in the situation, taking illness, baggage, anger, and past pain to your next life transition; that would be living in hell.

Release all past pain. You don't want to take your baggage with you into your next life or through your transition.

Imagine how good it feels leaving all baggage behind you and only walking in the Spirit, Love, and Joy of who you are; that's walking in Heaven.

Speaking the Language of Miracles reminds you of who you are.

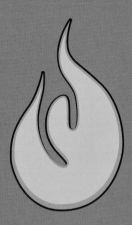

God says:

I AM VICTORIOUS THROUGH HIM WHO LOVES ME.

GOD GAVE US THE GIFT OF FREE CHOICE

ASK YOURSELF: ARE YOU USING YOUR GOD-GIVEN GIFTS?

When you apply this to
every part of your life:
"The situation is not who
I am," you allow your
God-given gifts that are
inside of you to rise up
and walk in Victory.
By not walking in the
situation you automatically
walk in the outcome of
what you want to achieve.

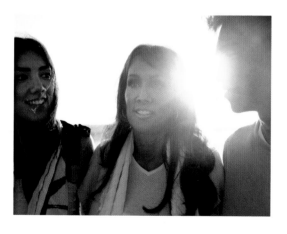

THANK YOU, GOD

About the Author

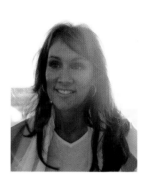

Your life can change in an instant. And you can intentionally change your life in an instant.

I've lived through the first statement multiple times, in ways I wouldn't wish on anyone. When I was 15 years old, I was pronounced dead at the scene of a horrific motorcycle accident. My husband was once told he had six months to live. When my son, Brandon, was 10 years old, he was diagnosed with a rare form of Leukemia and was told he wouldn't be leaving the hospital.

None of those events ever came to pass, if it wasn't for Speaking the Language of Miracles®. My walk has created in me, an intense knowing, that we have the ability to access the incredible power we are through our own language.

YOU ARE POWERFUL. WHAT IS INSIDE OF YOU, IS GREATER THAN ANY SITUATION.

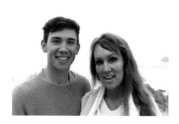

Our Vision with this book is to bring out and affirm Your Greatness. Discover yourself and celebrate who you are. You are the creator of your life. Create a life you love.

REMEMBER: THE SITUATION IS NOT WHO YOU ARE®

John L. Scott
F O U N D A T I O N

About the Foundation

The John L. Scott Foundation was founded in 1997 in honor of John L. Scott, a philanthropist and community activist who believed in the value of giving back. Participating in the Foundation is 100% voluntary. Our brokers who sign up give a portion out of each of their commissions, every time they have a home sale close. Our support also has the option to give out of each of their paychecks. We work with about 16 different hospitals and children's programs in Washington, Oregon, Idaho and California. Each one of our office is set up for their donations to benefit the children's hospital closest to them.

The mission of the The John L. Scott Foundation is supported by the generous donations and volunteer efforts of our sales associates and office support teams. These voluntary contributions enable the John L. Scott Foundation to help sponsor events that help raise millions of dollars for children's hospitals throughout the Pacific Northwest each year.

Twenty (20%) percent of the net proceeds from books sales of Speaking the Language of Miracles goes directly to support Children's Hospitals in the Pacific Northwest.

speakingthelanguageofmiracles.com